When the Storm Doesn't End:
God's Presence in the Midst of Chronic Pain

Reece B. Sherman

Why has my pain been perpetual
And my wound incurable, refusing
to be healed?
Will You indeed be to me like a
deceptive stream
With water that is
unreliable? (Jeremiah 15:18 NASB)

Table of Contents:

First Chapter: The Storm...A Parable

It began to rain softly. It came without warning. I wasn't expecting it...nor was I bothered by it. Rain comes and goes. It's a part of life. Some days it rains, other days it doesn't. Some days we experience a drizzle or a downpour. Other days are dry and hot. Still other days are windy or the snow falls softly.

Meteorology is not an exact science. Like life, we look for patterns and signs. History plays a small part, but each day is a new opportunity to discover just what the weather pattern will be. One TV meteorologist, Steve Pool, is quoted as saying: "I enjoy being a television forecaster. It's one of the few jobs that you can be absolutely dead wrong on a somewhat regular basis and remain employed." (***Watching Weather***, pg. 113).

This day the rain began without warning, but also without any call for concern. Rain is a part of nature's cycle. God ordained rain. It is needed to bring growth and cleansing. The schedule God set for nature is consistent and complete. God's creation needs rainfall and sunshine. It is a system of nourishment for the earth that God set at the time of creation.

So, on that day, when the rain began, I had no reason not to believe that in a matter of time the sun would push its way through the clouds and nature's cycle would be consistent. It would rain for a time and then it would end. I had no way of knowing that this rain was the beginning of a storm that would last and last.

I went inside. I stayed inside for the rest of the day. I had no real reason to go outside. To some the rain is calming. It brings a feeling of security...even God's presence. Some feel safe, with the rain outside and the warmth inside. To some all is well with the world when the soft rain begins to fall. The smell, the freshness, knowing that each plant is drinking up every drop...is reassuring...especially when you know that you can watch it from the comfort of being inside, dry and warm.

The rain continued to fall in the afternoon, which wasn't unusual. But I began to have the ominous feeling that this was a rain that had no thought of letting up. Harder and harder it came. And, although I was inside, I seemed to somehow feel the effects of it. The rumbles of thunder and flashes of lightning were somehow affecting both mind and body. And all I could do was waiting for it to pass. Pass...it didn't.

I walked to the window to watch the rain fall, to see if there was any sign of clearing. Then I noticed something that both amazed and puzzled me. There were children playing in the street. A neighbor walked her dog, obviously in no hurry. The world seemed to go on as usual. Couldn't they see that it was raining? I could feel each drop...why couldn't they? How were they able to stand outside amidst the blinding rain, the thunder and the flashes of lightning?

I felt almost like I was in a dream. I knew it was raining. I not only saw the rain, somehow I even felt the storm, yet, it seemed that I was the only one. My body shook with every rumble of thunder and I felt the shock of every flash of lightning. The world around me was going on as usual. Children were playing and laughing. Birds were singing in the trees. And the rain was falling harder and harder. Was I going crazy? I needed answers. I needed help.

"It's not raining and there is no reason for you to believe it is," was the first professional answer I heard. "The sky is blue, the sun is shining, and there is no storm." I left the weatherman's office bewildered...frustrated...and strangely alone. Weatherman after weatherman...the same answer, "No rain in sight."

But I felt the shock of every lightning bolt and my body quaked with the thunder. Every drop of rain found its target...me. It was almost as if I was living in an alternate world. Everyone else enjoyed the sunlight...and I stood alone in the rain. The storm makes you feel that way...alone. No one else feels what you feel, sees what you see, knows what you are going through. And you can't describe it.

Virginia Woolf wrote: "*The merest schoolgirl when she falls in love has [great writers and poets] to speak her mind for her, but let a sufferer try to describe his pain to a doctor and the language at once runs dry.*"

Even when you are surrounded by those who love you best, you feel a deep sense of aloneness. They can't feel your pain...not that you would want them to. Well, perhaps, for a few seconds...just so, for a moment, they know what you experience. Yes, probably one of the toughest parts of living in the storm is the feeling of being alone.

Oh...I know that I am not the only one living through a storm. There are many others like me. But the loneliness comes when you realize that there comes a point when you must quietly let the thunder shake you and the lightning strike you without a word. You must...or the words would flow continually. How do you convince someone of something they can't feel? How do you work through the

"It's all in your mind" comments from others? How do you live with a storm that doesn't end?

From the nights when the lightning flashes would jolt me awake to the days when I had to work and live in the middle of a downpour, I go on. I have been able to hide the never-ending storm from others.

It has been raining for close to 20 years now. I feel a little like Noah, wondering when the storm would stop and the waters would recede. At least Noah was warned that the storm was coming, and others witnessed the flooding rain. He also had time to prepare. And he knew it would end.

One of the first things I had to do was to tell myself that I wasn't crazy. I wasn't feeling something that wasn't there. It wasn't all in my mind. It was in my knees, elbows, shoulders, feet, toes, hands and fingers.

There were times when I felt that I found storm experts. They understand that the storm is very real. They just can't stop it. They have helped me know that I'm not crazy. They have also prescribed medications that turn the downpour into a drizzle at times. I am grateful for all that they can do.

I have also known that God has been aware of my storm all along. At times I have yelled for him to "Close the heavens and Stop the rain!" Other times have found me asking "Why?" And...there are times when I just ask him to help me to sleep during the storm.

I reflect on the time Jesus was able to sleep during the storm on the Sea of Galilee. Peaceful, restful sleep...while the disciples feared for their lives. When they woke him up and asked "Don't you care whether or not we die?" Jesus stilled the storm and told them that they had little faith. I would love to be able to sleep during the storm...like Jesus. I have often wondered if I can't because of lack of faith. I will talk more about that later. For now...I can say with confidence, both, that I live in the midst of a storm, and that I live with God.

Dr. Tom Murphree, professor of meteorology at the Naval Postgraduate School in Monterey, California describes a storm as "a violent and short-lived readjustment of the atmosphere toward a more stable condition. When cold air and warm air meet and start mixing it up, the natural tendency is for the relatively buoyant warm air to come to rest on top of the heavier cool air. That's the stable condition. Blizzards, hurricanes, thunderstorms and tornadoes are all part of the process of getting to that stable condition." (***Watching Weather***, by Tom Murphree and Mary K.

Miller, Henry Holt and Company, New York, 1998. page 77).

This book is about getting to a more stable condition. Although the storm may continue there is a way to find stability of spirit. As Murphree stated, a part of getting to that (more) stable condition includes blizzards, hurricanes, thunderstorms and tornadoes. He says that the violence of the weather is needed to bring about stability. Whatever the result, the "violence" of the storm can have a tremendous effect on us.

Chapter Two: The Effects of the Storm (synopsis)

"Unrelieved pain has enormous physiological and psychological effects on patients," says Dennis S. O'Leary, MD, President of the Joint Commission on Accreditation of Healthcare Organizations (JACHO).

"We've all heard it before: 'It's in your head.' The truth is that all chronic pain has both the physiological and psychological components. The diagnostic problem is to assess the relative contribution of these components on your experience of pain. Nevertheless, there is a persistent tendency to ignore or deny the psychological component of pain because of either fear or misinformation. In fact, chronic pain often induces psychological factors." (<u>The Effects of Chronic Pain</u>, Dr. Timothy K. Quek, HomePage, 7/30/02).

Living in the storm that never ends can affect an individual in many ways. It has the capacity to:

1. **Dampen the spirit**

Attitude is everything...or so they say. If that is the case...the storm has a way of taking ones spirit to the depths. It can seep into the mind and heart of the chronic pain sufferer and wash away hope, and joy, and strength.

Jeremiah wrote in Lamentations 1:12: *"Is it nothing to you, all you who pass by? Look around and see. Is any suffering like my suffering that was inflicted on me, that the LORD brought on me in the day of his fierce anger?"* Jeremiah has a lot of company in lamenting about his pain.

Chronic pain often brings with it a woeful spirit. Because of the pain, the feeling of no end in sight, and the failure of physicians to bring about a "cure", a general melancholic feeling is common. The desire to seek joy is affected. The desire to do anything is affected. Too many times, there is a "woe is me" attitude that shows its ugly head. This, in effect, results in inhibitions to seek social events. And it, therefore, may affect relationships.

2. **Muddy the Pathway**

Part of dealing with chronic pain is questioning the right path to take. The storm muddies the path. It is difficult to know which way to turn and who to turn to. It is especially difficult if the path you have taken has led to dead-ends.

I know firsthand the experience of not knowing which way to turn. There was no clear path. My problem was that I wanted a doctor to give me quick relief. They didn't...and couldn't. In fact many could not give me a reason for my pain. Therefore I had no place to turn, the path before me was muddied.

3. **Cloud the Vision**

The storm is often blinding. The rain is so intense that you can only see the storm. You cannot see the people around you. You pay no attention to the world of nature. You are blinded to the good that is in your life. The world has a gray hue. Everything is colored by the pain that is experienced.

4. **Erode Confidence**

Confidence in what can be done to gain help. When nothing has helped after so many doctor visits, hope for relief erodes. Confidence in what others...medical professionals, can do diminishes until it is almost gone. Although I will say that **there is usually a strong desire to keep looking for an answer...because the pain won't let you give up**.

Confidence in what the sufferer can do without getting

<u>hurt</u>. There is a hesitancy to do physical work that may cause more pain. Exercise programs have a sense of fear attached to them. This is a problem, because often it is a proper exercise regimen that may be a major help to many who suffer from chronic pain. But the fear of causing more pain keeps many from proper exercise.

5. **Flood the Mind**

Chronic pain is frustrating. Scott Fishman tells us that "**Chronic pain Can become an emotion as strong as hatred or love and can dominate your every thought and action**." (*The War on Pain,* pg. 66).

I cannot tell you how many times I am involved in a worship program or watching a television show, or doing something else...and the pain hits me. Then **IT** becomes my focus. It floods my mind. It demands attention. I am in a profession where I need to pay attention to the people I am helping. I feel that I do a good job of that. But there are times when my pain wants to dominate my thoughts. My knee or finger will shout out "Don't forget about me!"

6. **Reveal the Cracks**

My parents say that I was accident-prone as a child. I now know better after years of therapy. I was abused as a child. I have had stitches in my head more times than I can remember. Every now and then I'll put my hand on my scalp and notice blood on my hand. Maybe there are still some open places that didn't completely close, because the storm has often found a way to seep into the cracks.

I am speaking metaphorically more than literally. When one suffers from chronic pain, the cracks are often emotional,

psychological, even attitudinal.
There are places that we have open
wounds. There are areas where we
are not completely healed. There
are problems that we have not
dealt with properly and we have left
an opening for the storm to seep
in.
These cracks may be found in our:
- attitudes
- faith
- psychological weaknesses
- old wounds
- personality problems
- etc...

7. **Affect Activities**:
As I mentioned earlier,
chronic pain can be very limiting. It
can cause us to go into a shell. The
storm is often easier to deal with
when we don't have to go "outside"
into the world. There is safety
staying at home.
This, of course, brings with it
many social implications, especially

when your work has to do with being with people. Without God's help, the difficulty would be so much greater. I have also found that everyone has problems and pains that they deal with. This has given me a desire to minister to them. Often I find that I am ministered to in return.

Finally, the Storm will:

8. **Test the Strength of One's Foundation**

In Matthew 7:24-27 (which I will deal with in more detail in chapter four), Jesus speaks of the man who built his house upon the rock and the man who built on sand. The house built on the rock stood through the storm. The house built on the sand did not.

The storm has a way of testing the strength of one's foundation. Especially one's faith foundation. The storm tests one's faith in God and in his ability or desire to help.

If the foundation is not secure...the storm of chronic pain can bring about a tremendous amount of damage to one's life. Really, it is one's faith foundation that makes the difference in the ability to cope...the ability to survive.

Chapter Three: The Storm - Chronic Pain - My Story

According to Joann Ellison Rodgers, in *Drugs & Pain*, there **are four components of pain**:

1. **First**, the nervous system detects damage to some tissue.
2. **Second**, the perception of the pain itself which causes certain chemicals to be released at the site of the injury and elsewhere.
3. **Third**, our reaction to the pain. "This is when suffering begins. At

this point the person usually reacts with a yell, tears, fear, anxiety, or depression"

4. **Fourth**, and finally, is what John D. Loeser of the University of Washington in Seattle calls "Pain Behavior." This, he says, is "anything a person says or does or does not do that would lead one to infer that a [painful] stimulus has occurred." (*Drugs and Pain*, by Joann Ellison Rodgers, from <u>The Encyclopedia of Psychoactive Drugs</u>, Series 2. Solomon H. Snyder, M.D., General Editor, Chelsea House Publishers, New York, New Haven, Philadelphia, 1987. PP. 29-33).

Pain is a part of life. Chronic pain controls life. It affects every decision...every thought...every movement. Chronic pain must always be acknowledged. It demands it. Some sufferers deal with it every moment. Others live anticipating when it will deal with them.

Acute pain is different. It usually comes on rapidly, and lasts for a shorter duration...much like a bee sting. Although acute pain can become chronic pain, chronic pain is different, it usually comes on gradually and worsens. It lasts for a longer duration, sometimes for the lifetime of the sufferer. It is like a storm that doesn't end. It can become disabling. At the very least, it is a constant source of aggravation and frustration.

Chronic pain interferes with the lives of more than thirty-five million American adults (***Your Pain Is Real***, Emile Hiesiger with Kathleen Brady, 2001, Regan Books, HarperCollins, New York, In the Forward by John D. Loeser, M.D. pg. xiii). Although many people experience chronic pain, it is an individual experience. No one feels my pain. No one feels your pain. Each person's experience is unique... personal.

Pain is a mind-body experience. It affects both thought and emotion. "The common thoughts and emotions in people dealing with chronic pain: The emotions include: anger/rage, anxiety, depression, fear, grief and mourning, guilt, hostility, shame, and remembered pain. Thoughts include: abandonment, alienation, dependency, disease and death, future, loss, mental illness, and past." (***Medical, Psychological and Vocational Aspects of Disability***, eds. Martin G. Brodwin, Fernando A. Tellez, and Sandra K. Brown. Revised printing, 1995. Elliot & Fitzpatrick, Inc., Athens, GA. pg. 185).

My own personal storm came in the form of RSDS - Reflex Sympathetic Dystrophy Syndrome. It is also referred to as CRPS - Complex Regional Pain Syndrome.

Basically it is a disorder of the Sympathetic Nervous System. There is still some mystery surrounding all that is involved in RSDS. It is a painful disorder. It reminds me daily of my humanness with its burning, knife-like, shooting pain.

It began after my first of three knee surgeries. The 2nd and 3rd surgical procedures were meant to relieve the pain...instead they made the pain more severe and permanent. It has since spread to other joints. There is nothing structurally wrong with me...but my brain believes there is...therefore the lightning shoots through my body daily.

As a minister I walk (gingerly) among people who understand chronic pain and also live with it on a daily basis. One lady in my weekly Bible study class suffers with fibromyalgia, a condition that causes muscle pain and tenderness as well as other complications. She suffers constant pain and the medication she has been prescribed causes hallucinations, so she can't take it.

Another church member, a man in his nineties, suffers with severe back pain and has endured countless surgeries and treatments. He has lived a long, active life. One of the best fishermen I have ever known. Spent the last days of his life bedridden. His will was strong...but pain was his constant companion.

It takes courage to live with chronic pain. Courage and help. Courage and understanding. Courage and faith. Courage alone isn't enough. All the courage and determination in the world isn't enough to handle the storm that doesn't end.

The help of a family who understands and sympathizes is

vital. Realizing that it isn't easy living with a person who suffers chronic pain. But to face it alone would be unbearable. Having understanding family and friends is very important.

We need the help of doctors who understand our particular condition. It often takes long hours and many office visits to find a physician who can understand and help. Physicians can't "cure" every condition. In my particular situation, the physicians who tried to "cure" me actually made my condition worse. And then without admitting their limitations told me that I wasn't in pain. It was all in my head. I have since found wonderful medical care.

We need the help of God. I'm not listing help from God here because it is lower on the scale of needs or because asking for God's help is a last resort. It isn't. God's help should be our first desire.

However, there is something about living with chronic pain that has a way of affecting one's relationship with God. Often the relationship suffers, at least in the beginning. **The question "Why? is a constant cry**. When we ask for God's healing and it doesn't come...our faith is tested.

In ***The War on Pain***, Scott Fishman states: "Perhaps one of the most eloquent thinkers to delve into the nature of suffering is Viktor Frankl, a psychiatrist who survived a Nazi concentration camp and wrote in his seminal work, ***Man's Search for Meaning***. Early in the book, he recounts his reaction to a guard beating him. 'At such a moment, it is not the physical pain which hurts the most...it is the mental agony caused by the injustice, the unreasonableness of it all.' Pain forces you to keep asking 'Why me?' yet there is no answer." (***The War on Pain***, by Scott

Fishman, M.D. with Lisa Berger. HarperCollins, 2000, New York, NY. page 16).

On the other hand...living in a storm that doesn't end has a way of building a much stronger relationship with the only one who can truly help. There is constant leaning on God. There is a daily prayer for strength and stamina. There is the wonderful feeling that you have made it through the day but without God's help you wouldn't have.

Chapter Four: The Scriptures and the Storm

The Scriptures are full of references to the rain and the storm and God's Lordship over their beginning, ending and effects. From the time of creation God has been Lord over the wind, rain and lightning. He brings the thunderous storm and the gentle rain.

Often the storm is written of in its reality. There are other times when the metaphor of rain and storm describe the experiences of mankind or the individual. The Psalmist especially likes to refer to his experiences as well as the experiences of God's people by using the metaphor of a storm. In Psalm 135:7, he states: *He causes the clouds to ascend from the ends of the earth;*
Who makes lightnings for the rain, Who brings forth the wind from His treasuries.

Let's discover several passages that refer to the rain and storm, both literally and metaphorically and its effects upon the earth and her inhabitants:

- **Genesis 7:12** - *And rain fell on the earth forty days and forty nights...*

This was the experience of Noah and those who lived during his day. The rain fell and fell and seemed that it would never stop. Although God told Noah that the rain would end after forty days. In other words, Noah was assured of an ending time for the rain.

The storm came in order to cleanse the earth of the sinfulness of mankind. God was beginning anew. He was starting over. He was seeking to bring back that which he had desired from the beginning...a people who would trust him and worship him as Lord of their lives. **The storm came for a reason**.

However, even the faithful ones, Noah and his family were affected by the storm. The rain ended after forty days, but they had no idea how long it would take for the waters to subside.

The Lord kept the faithful safe during the storm. He kept his promise. He brought about the cleansing he desired and he kept Noah and his family safe during the rain of judgment.

- **Deuteronomy 32:2** - *Let my teaching fall like rain and my words descend like dew, like showers on new grass, like abundant rain on tender plants.*

The writer of Deuteronomy speaks of God's teaching as rain falling on the earth. The rain is used as a symbol of God's precepts falling gently upon his people. There is a serenity to this passage. **God's lessons do not always have to be learned the hard way. If we are open, the gentle rain can teach us what we need to know to travel life's**

road. Perhaps it is because we fail to learn from the gentle rain that God must send the storm.

- **2 Chronicles 6:26-27** - *"When the heavens are shut up and there is no rain because they have sinned against You, and they pray toward this place and confess Your name, and turn from their sin when You afflict them; then hear in heaven and forgive the sin of Your servants and Your people Israel, indeed, teach them the good way in which they should walk. And send rain on Your land which You have given to Your people for an inheritance.*

These words are part of the glorious prayer of Solomon at the dedication of the Temple. Here it is the lack of rain that is seen as judgment that God uses on his people. It is designed to bring about prayer and obedience. This is not the only place in Scripture where lack of rain is used as a warning to turn to god. We remember the story of Elijah and his dealings with King Ahab and Queen Jezebel when the rain was held back for three years.

One gets the feeling that the lack of rain represents the silence of God. The heavens are quiet. There is no communication...no active relationship with mankind. **You come away with the question as to which is worse, the rain or the silent heavens**.

Now we turn to the Psalmist who often spoke of the storm and the rain to magnify the Lordship of God over the earth.

Psalm 29: 3-11 - *The voice of the Lord is upon the waters; The God of glory thunders, the Lord is over* *many waters. The voice of the Lord is powerful, the voice of the Lord is majestic. The voice of the Lord breaks the cedars; Yes, the Lord breaks in pieces the cedars of Lebanon. He makes Lebanon skip like a calf, and Sirion like a young wild ox. The voice of the Lord hews out lightning (like flames) of fire, The voice of the Lord shakes the wilderness; the Lord shakes the wilderness of Kadesh. The voice of the Lord makes the deer to calve and strips the forests bare; and in his temple everything says, "Glory!" The Lord sat as King at the flood; Yes, the Lord sits as King forever. The Lord will give strength to his people; The Lord will bless his people with peace.*

Throughout this Psalm, the "voice" of the Lord is seen as the driving force behind the storm. And **his voice is heard above the storm**. Through the thunder and the lightning, God's voice is heard. Through the breaking of the cedars and the rising waves, the Lord can still be heard. It is almost as if the storm is sent to get the people's attention and then they are to listen to the louder and more forceful voice that rises above the storm. **It is a reminder that God speaks through even the greatest storms of life. And it also brings about the truth that God often needs to get our attention before we are at the point where we can hear his voice and learn from him.**

This is not a gentle rain. The Psalmist describes a storm of mighty proportions. But the Lord is not absent as the thunder shakes the ground and the lightning like "flames of fire" shoots from the heavens. He is the Lord of the storm. He is the Lord of life. He "sits enthroned over the flood."

Then the Psalmist includes a prayer for peace...peace in the midst of the storm.

Psalm 107: 23-31 - *Some went down to the sea in ships, doing business on the mighty waters; they saw the deeds of the LORD, his wondrous works in the deep. For he commanded and raised the stormy wind, which lifted up the waves of the sea. They mounted up to heaven, they went down to the depths; their courage melted away in their calamity; they reeled and staggered like drunkards, and were at their wits' end. Then they cried to the LORD in their trouble, and he brought them out from their distress; he made the storm be still, and the waves of the sea were hushed. Then they were glad because they had quiet, and he brought them to their desired haven. Let them thank* *the LORD for his steadfast love, for his wonderful works to humankind.*

Here again, we find God sending a storm intended to teach a lesson. We have courageous seafarers who lean on their own expertise and bravery to deal with the deep. God sends a storm and then they are forced to cry to him...realizing that he is their strength. All the courage and knowledge of the deep could not keep them safe through the storm they encountered. Some fail to realize that truth. These men didn't. They turned to God for help and he calmed the storm and brought them into the harbor safely.

Now, words from the prophet Isaiah:

Isaiah 30:19-23 - *Truly, O people in Zion, inhabitants of Jerusalem, you shall weep no more. He will* *surely be gracious to you at the sound of your cry; when he hears it, he will answer you. Though the Lord may give you the bread of adversity and the water of affliction, yet your Teacher will not hide himself any more, but your eyes shall see your Teacher. And when you turn to the right or when you turn to the left, your ears shall hear a word behind you, saying, "This is the way; walk in it." Then you will defile your silver-covered idols and your gold-plated images. You will scatter them like filthy rags; you will say to them, "Away with you!" He will give rain for the seed with which you sow the ground, and grain, the produce of the ground, which will be rich and plenteous. On that day your cattle will graze in broad pastures.*

These are words of hope for the people who suffered exile from their home. Isaiah reminded them that God had not forgotten them. Yes, they were suffering through difficulty because of their own sin. Yes, God himself sent calamity on them. But he had not forgotten them.

They were called to turn to him. The affliction they were facing could only be changed by turning to God for help. Then they could be assured a future where God would send rain...rain that would bring newness and life and growth.

Isaiah 55:10-11 - *"For as the rain and the snow come down from heaven, And do not return there without watering the earth; And making it bear and sprout, And furnishing seed to the sower and bread to the eater;*
So will My word be which goes forth from My mouth; It will not return to Me empty, without accomplishing what I desire, And without

succeeding in the matter for which I sent it."

This is probably one of the most familiar Old Testament passages concerning rain. It reminds us that the rain is sent for a purpose. It is designed to bring about growth. It is designed to bring about life. **God sends the rain and the word. Often he sends them at the same time. They are both designed to accomplish God's purpose.**

Directly before this passage are the words, *"For as the heavens are higher than the earth, so are My ways higher than your ways; And My thoughts than your thoughts."*(v.9)

One cannot explain the ways of God. **Sometimes the hard rain comes without warning. Sometimes the word comes bringing correction and discipline. Sometimes the rain**

falls softly and the word is gentle. Whatever the form and the intensity, they come for a purpose that God wants to accomplish.

The New Testament also uses the metaphors of rain and storms to teach life lessons.

In the Sermon on the Mount we read: *He* (God) *causes his sun to rise on the evil and the good, and sends rain on the righteous and the unrighteous* (**Matthew 5:45**).

What an important lesson! **Good and bad come to both the good and the bad**. Sun and rain fall upon both the righteous and the unrighteous. The calm and the storm, the peaceful and the perilous, come to all. The Bible doesn't promise life without rain to the righteous. He doesn't promise that we will always enjoy sunny days. When calamity falls on the evil we say "They deserved what happened...they deserved the storm." But when it comes our way we ask "Why?"

Often we forget the love that God has for all his creatures. And we also seem to forget that the difference between the righteous and unrighteous is not one of experience as much as it is one of how one deals with the experiences that comes one's way. That is the lesson found later in the Sermon on the Mount in **Matthew 7:24-27**: *"Therefore everyone who hears these words of Mine and acts on them, may be compared to a wise man who built his house on the rock. And the rain fell, and the[c] floods came, and the winds blew and slammed against that house; and yet it did not fall, for it had been founded on the rock. Everyone who hears these words of Mine and does not act on them, will be like a foolish man who* *built his house on the sand. The rain fell, and the floods came, and the winds blew and slammed against that house; and it fell—and great was its fall."*

Storms come to the wise and the foolish, the righteous and the unrighteous. **The affect they have upon our lives is up to us and our relationship with the Lord of the storm**. That is the message of Scripture. God is the Lord of the storm. The storm will come. Some suffer through it for longer than expected. Sometimes the end of the storm isn't anywhere in sight. **But knowing God is the Lord of it...should make a tremendous difference. It is only when we acknowledge that, that we are able to feel his presence in the midst of it and hear his voice over it**.

Chapter Five: Living and Learning in the Storm

Three Stings
George got stung by a bee and
said,
"I wouldn't have got stung if I'd
stayed in bed."
Fred got stung and we heard him
roar,
"What am I being punished for?"
Lew got stung and we heard him
say,
"I learned somethin' about bees
today." (author unknown)

"Pain is a teacher, the
headmaster of nature's survival
school, and like any teacher it
requires pupils with the ability to
learn." (***Why We Hurt*: The
Natural History of Pain**, by Frank
T. Vertosick, Jr., M.D. Harcourt, Inc.

New York, San Diego, London. 2000. pg. 2). Pain is a teacher, and learning must take place. Just like the Scriptural references to the storm and rain, there are lessons to be learned.

A lady in a former church once made the statement to me that my preaching had gotten better since my knee started hurting. At the time I didn't fully appreciate the statement, although I accepted it graciously. But now I have more insight into what she meant. When life is good and easy, it is difficult to understand those who do not experience life that same way.   That does not mean that ministers who have not experienced chronic suffering cannot preach to meet the needs of their people. God has a way, if we listen to him, of placing the right minister in the right congregation. It does, however, mean that even those who minister without personal experience of chronic pain must know their people and live with them in their pain, in order to understand them and speak life-changing words to them.

In twenty years I have seen at least twenty doctors, six physical therapists, three massage therapists, and four psychologists. I have gone through eight surgeries, two cryofreeze procedures, twelve acupuncture treatments, electrical stimulation, and have been prescribed most, if not all, medications that can be prescribed for my conditions.

The storm still rages. So what have I learned? Or, better yet, what am I learning?

I am learning that I am part of the world around me. What do I mean by that? I mean that I am no better off, no different than those who walk with me or by me each day. I have no immunity from the cares and concerns, the problems and pains that others face, Being a Christian does not keep me from facing storms.

However, Faith in the Lord of the storm means that I have a foundation, a rock-hard foundation, that will keep me from crumbling when the storm blows. Faith in God and faith in what God can or will do are different...at least for me.

My faith is stronger than ever. I trust him to be present and to give me strength. He watches me and makes a way for me to make it through each day. Doubting God's existence or his love are not thoughts that fill my days.

I also have faith in God's healing power. Although some may doubt that I have enough faith since I have not experienced God's physical healing. I do truly believe that God can heal me. I believe that he can make the storm end. He can calm the storm that has lasted for so long. I believe God has healed others from chronic afflictions. I believe in a God who can heal...a God who can take away pain. **My struggle is not whether or not I have faith that God can heal, but whether or not he will heal**.

According to Frank T. Vertosick, Jr., M.D. "In his book , **_The Problem of Pain_**, theologian C.S. Lewis...argues that God could never command our attention if we lived in an anesthetic world....If Lewis is correct, God has the power to create a pain-free existence but will not do so out of fear of being rendered unneeded, ignored, and irrelevant." (*Why We Hurt*, pg. 9)

Some may read that statement and believe that it paints a picture of a weak and insecure God. Others may say that God is cruel. I read the statement and see some biblical basis for it. As I reflected in Chapter Three, Scripture bears out the truth that God teaches us lessons through the storms. One of the most important lessons that we learn is that we cannot...or should not live life apart from a relationship with God.

I do not believe that God is insecure and brings pain into our lives to keep us from living our lives without needing his assistance. I do, however, believe that God is our Creator and he demands our acknowledgement. And, yes, there are times when we may not acknowledge God if life was easy.

Let me say at this point that **I do not believe that every pain that we face or feel comes from God**. Some pain comes from our own actions. Some comes from the actions of others. Some comes because someone who was drunk decided to get behind the wheel of a car. Some comes from carelessness. However the pain comes...God must be acknowledged because he wants to help us face days that would be unbearable otherwise.

There is an old story about an atheist who had an old tree in his backyard. During a storm the tree fell on his neighbor's house. The atheist called his insurance company to see if he was covered. His insurance agent was a good, churchgoing man and knew about the atheist's lack of belief. With this in mind, he gave the following response to the atheist: "If your tree fell over because it was dead, we cannot cover this expense; you will have to pay the repairs on your neighbor's home yourself. However, if the tree fell because of "an act of God" your insurance will cover it. So which one do you consider it to be?" (Heavenward, *Stories for Preachers and Teachers*).
There comes a time when we should acknowledge God's presence in the midst of the storm. There comes a time when we should

realize that there is a power and a presence that is greater than our pain.

Suffering is viewed as both a curse and a blessing in Scripture. In many places God brings about suffering as a punishment upon the wicked and disobedient. Even his own people are not immune. In these verses, suffering is something to be avoided:

Romans 1:18 - *For the wrath of God is revealed from heaven against all ungodliness and unrighteousness of men who suppress the truth in unrighteousness.*
Psalm 119:67 - *Before I was afflicted I went astray, but now I obey our word.*

In other biblical passages, suffering is something to be pursued. It is seen as a blessing. It is a way of identifying and sharing in the sufferings of Christ.

Philippians 1:29-30 - *For it has been granted to you on behalf of Christ not only to believe on him, but also to suffer for him, since you are going through the same struggle you saw I had, and now hear that I still have.*
1 Peter 4:13 - *"...to the degree that you share in the sufferings of Christ, keep on rejoicing."*

In still other places, suffering is seen as something that occurs simply because of our humanness. It is something from which we pray to God for relief. **James 5:13** reads, *"...is anyone suffering? Let him pray."*

In some places suffering is brought about by lack of faith...or seen as a result of little faith. In other places suffering is considered as a necessary step to greater faith.

Romans 5:3-5 - *And not only this, but we also exult in our tribulations, knowing that tribulation brings about perseverance; and perseverance, proven character; and proven character, hope; and hope does not disappoint, because the love of God has been poured out within our hearts through the Holy Spirit who was given to us.*

This is what Paul is saying:

Suffering >
Perseverance >
Character >
Hope >
An Understanding of God's Love.

Suffering teaches us things that we could not learn otherwise. **It's like taking an egg and dropping it in boiling water...it becomes hard. But if you take a potato and do the same...it becomes soft. We can**

respond to our suffering by becoming hardened to life and to God. Or we can respond by becoming soft and teachable. If we respond like the potato...suffering can teach us great lessons.

1 Peter 1:6-7 - *In this you greatly rejoice, even though now for a little while, if necessary, you have been distressed by various trials, so that the proof of your faith, being more precious than gold which is perishable, even though tested by fire, may be found to result in praise and glory and honor at the revelation of Jesus Christ.*

Theologian Malcolm Muggeridge reflecting on his life said: "Contrary to what might be expected, I look back on experiences that at the time seemed especially desolating and painful with particular satisfaction. Indeed, I can say with complete truthfulness that everything I have learned in my 75 years in this world, everything that has truly enhanced and enlightened my experience, has been through affliction and not through happiness."

Billy Graham, in his book, ***Till Armageddon*** wrote: "These words were found penned on the wall of a prison cell in Europe: 'I believe in love even when I don't feel it. I believe in God even when he is silent.' "

Therefore we must ask ourselves, "Just who is in control here?" Is Marcel Proust right when he said, "Illness is the doctor to who we pay the most heed. To kindness, to knowledge, we make promises only. Pain we obey."

Those who live with chronic pain know that there is a constant battle for control of our thoughts, emotions, schedules, and actions. **That which is in control dictates what we do, rules our relationships, and governs our general attitude toward life**.

When pain is in control, I have difficulty being around too many people. I would rather be alone. I will often crawl in bed and try to sleep until the pain subsides. Oftentimes pain wakes me from sleep. I have been told that I cry out in pain during my sleep. However, when pain is in control it is of my choosing. **Being in pain doesn't mean that I have to allow it to control me**. Oh...it may control the way I walk, or IF I walk. But it doesn't need to control my attitude 100% of the time. The pain I face doesn't come and go...it simply intensifies or lessens. It is a constant...but it doesn't have to control me. Although I will have to admit that it sometimes does.

Emily Dickinson understood the control of pain when she wrote. **"The Mystery of Pain"**:

Pain has an element of blank;
It cannot recollect
When it began, or if there were
A day when it was not.
It has no future but itself,
Its infinite realms contain
Its past, enlightenment to perceive
New periods of pain.

The question is whether the storm itself or the Lord of the Storm is in control. There are **biblical principles to help us to make sure the Lord of the Storm is in control of our daily, although painful, existence**. Let me list them and then explain them:

1. **Acknowledge God's Presence**
2. **Accept His Presence**
3. **Acknowledge God's Lordship**
4. **Accept His Lordship**

5. **Make this acknowledgment and acceptance a ritual**: both day and night. This will be a constant reminder that:
a. **We are not alone**
b. **We nor our circumstances are in control**.

Proverbs 3:5-6 is the key verse to guide us in acknowledging and accepting God's presence and His Lordship:
Trust in the Lord with all thine heart; and lean not unto thine own understanding. In all thy ways acknowledge him, and he shall direct thy paths. (I use the familiar KJV).

It all begins with trust. In order to place God in control of our lives, we must trust him. We must trust that he cares. We must trust that he wants to help us. We must trust that he understands.

In his book, ***The Spiritual Life of Children***, Robert Coles Pulitzer Prize winning author and professor at Harvard University, tells of being in a classroom with 4th graders. He asked each one to draw a picture of God. Coles said that he had accumulated 293 pictures of God. He has found that you learn much about what children think of God by their drawings of him.

"That day in the classroom a young girl named Betsy expressed reluctance to draw God. She said 'When God came here, he looked like a man, he was Jesus. But then he went back to being God, and I don't know what he looks like now, but you have to have a face!' She proceeded to give him one... a big orange circle then wavy hair, and a neck at which point she abruptly stopped. She kept her left hand on the drawing paper. She had put the orange crayon down after finishing the neck...but couldn't decide what to do next. Finally she said 'It's a guess. I don't know if I'm on the right track. I'm not sure I should finish." Coles told her "It is a guess. There's no correct answer...only you and me with our paper and crayons.' Then Betsy said softly, 'I'll just do what I do,' as she began give the face eyes, a mouth and a nose. After giving God a full beard she sat and look at the picture she had done.

After a few fidgety moments the fourth-grader look out the window and said 'The clouds are coming. It may rain before school is out.' There was silence for a few seconds, then the question, 'Do you think God gets rained on?' Then after a few moments she answered her own question 'I think he gets rained on a lot...I know that when Jesus lived here he went through rainy days.' "

The Son of God was not immune to the storms. The Son of God understands.

Renew Me with Your Joy

When life's troubled waters

    Beat against my troubled heart,

Renew me with your joy, Dear Lord, and keep me close to you.

When the wind blows with vengeance

    And I find it difficult to stand,

Renew me with your joy, Dear Lord, and keep me close to you.

When the rains descend upon me

    And I cannot see your way,

Renew me with your joy, Dear
Lord, and keep me close to you.

When the ground beneath my feet

    Begins to shake my faith in You,

Renew me with your joy, Dear
Lord, and keep me close to you.

Your joy can calm the waters and
cause the winds to cease.

Your joy can clear the skies and fill
my heart with peace.

The storms of life can't harm me,
Lord

    If this one thing I do,

Renew me with your joy, Dear
Lord, and keep me close to you.

                    - Reece B. Sherman